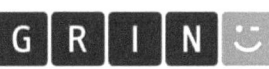

Bibliographic information published by the German National Library:

The German National Library lists this publication in the National Bibliography; detailed bibliographic data are available on the Internet at http://dnb.dnb.de .

Imprint:

Copyright © 2015 GRIN Verlag, Open Publishing GmbH
Print and binding: Books on Demand GmbH, Norderstedt Germany
ISBN: 9783668352681

This book at GRIN:

http://www.grin.com/en/e-book/345046/understanding-the-ebola-response-in-west-africa-utility-of-the-speech

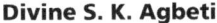

Divine S. K. Agbeti

Understanding the Ebola Response in West Africa. Utility of the "Speech Act" Discourse of Securitisation

GRIN Publishing

GRIN - Your knowledge has value

Since its foundation in 1998, GRIN has specialized in publishing academic texts by students, college teachers and other academics as e-book and printed book. The website www.grin.com is an ideal platform for presenting term papers, final papers, scientific essays, dissertations and specialist books.

Understanding the Ebola Response in West Africa: Utility of the 'Speech Act' Discourse of Securitisation

Author: Divine S. K. Agbeti

Table of Contents

Table of Figures

Appendices

Introduction

The alarming threats of infectious diseases, *inter alia*, anthrax, swine flu, Hantavirus, SARS, AIDS, and Ebola, have called for the concept of security to be redefined to include issues of infectious diseases and health, relevant to challenges that bedevil post-Cold War states. This has provided impetus to the emergence of health security and human security paradigms following the first United Nations Security Council's special session dedicated to AIDS. Subsequently, Canada and Denmark, among others, have explicitly included health security and human security issues in their national and foreign policies. Yet, traditional security scholars rebuff the idea of reconceptualising security to include health and infectious diseases, claiming that any alteration dilutes the meaning of security and renders "it a catch all term for anything negative" (Youde, 2004, p. 193). This research seeks to investigate how critical security scholars, particularly the Copenhagen School, contribute to our understanding of security in International Relations. Focusing on securitisation of health, the study draws on the recent Ebola pandemic in Guinea, Liberia, and Sierra Leone to explain the limitations of securitisation theory, propounded by the Copenhagen School, for International Relations theory.

The study argues that the Copenhagen School's conceptualisation of global security tends to favour a 'negative' version of security, fathomed as security from existential threats, supporting the traditional notion of security as survival. This isolates health issues from their systemic causes, instigating responsive mechanisms rather than preventative policies. Accordingly, substantial attention and resources are directed towards communicable, rather than non-communicable and chronic, diseases. The study also claims that this way of conceptualising security conjures the understanding of health via the prism of state interests, as pandemic and communicable diseases are perceived to pose potential threats to state security. Thus, securitisation practice bequeaths priority to state security over human security, and therefore fails to tackle the structural causes of global health inequalities that produce and reproduce these pandemics.

This study is divided into two parts: the first critically analyses the theoretical framework of securitisation. It methodically examines securitisation assumptions of Barry Buzan, Jaap de Wilde and Ole Waever (1998); the strengths of the securitisation framework, particularly in securitising health; and limitations of the securitisation theory to understanding global health issues. These analyses set the context for the second part of the study, 'Ebola case study in West Africa - Guinea, Liberia, and Sierra Leone'. The Ebola case study particularly demonstrates that global health issues only become security priorities when Western countries feel threatened, most especially when coined as a national security threat to the US and the UK.

Speech Act Discourse and Securitisation

Buzan et al.'s (1998) seminal work, *Security: a new framework of analysis*, adopted a 'speech act' approach to security study, broadening the security agenda to include threats beyond traditional state-centric and military conceptions of security. To include individuals, sub-state groups, and global concerns such as the environment that were marginalised by the traditional notion of security, Buzan et al. (also known as the Copenhagen School) developed a distinct perspective in the security debate, treating security as a social process outcome, rather than an objective condition. This inter-subjective nature of representing social issues as security threats is performed by securitising 'speech acts', grounded on J. L. Austin's speech act theory, which argued language is not only used to describe or convey a meaning but also to constitute a form of action or a social activity (Austin, 1962; Buzan, Waever, & de Wilde, 1998). For instance, a speaker saying "thank you," "you are fired" or "I nominate," is employing "language not just for the purposes of description, but also for actually doing something else with wider social significance – hence the term speech acts" (Elbe, 2010, p. 11). Subsequently, constructing who or what is being secured, and from what, develops from a securitising speech act through which a particular threat becomes represented and recognised (Williams, 2003, p. 513). This implies that there are choices involved in deciding which issues are to be labelled as security threats.

According to Buzan et al. (1998, pp. 26-36), a security speech act comprises five integral elements to be met for a successful securitisation to occur: securitising actors, referent objects, existential threat, a call for emergency measures, and audience. Securitising actors such as political leaders and intelligence experts must declare a referent object such as a state, society, or population, to be existentially threatened (Elbe, 2010, p. 11; Williams, 2003). The securitising actors must then make a persuasive appeal to implement emergency measures to counter the existential threat (Elbe, 2010, p. 11; Williams, 2003); and the audience must sufficiently accept the claim for political actions to be taken that would not have otherwise been conceivable in a routine political setting (Elbe, 2010, p. 11; Williams, 2003). Governments, international organisations, and non-governmental organisations contend that the survival of state, communities, or individuals is highly at risk, unless desperate measures are taken by national and international actors to avert those crucial threats. Accordingly, health security, environmental security, and food security have been advanced with the linguistic grammar of security speech acts.

While scholars argue conceptualising health security debates as the securitisation of 'health' (Youde, 2004; Elbe, 2010), the question arises whether health securitisation can bypass the restraints of regular politics. In answer, Waever (1995) maintains that "the use of security label does not merely reflect whether a problem is a security problem, it is also a political choice, that is, a decision to conceptualise in a special way" (p. 65). For example, political parties in the UK choose whether to represent immigration issues as a security threat or as a human rights concern. Likewise, policy elites in international organisations choose whether to characterise health issues as public, development, or international security concerns. The ensuing paragraphs analyse the strengths and limitations of the Copenhagen School.

Strengths and Limitations of Copenhagen School

The Copenhagen School's securitisation theory has added greatly to our understanding of security in international relations. Buzan et al. (1998) have broadened the security agenda to include referent objects marginalised by the traditional conception of security. While the traditional notion of security focuses on military threats, the Copenhagen School successfully argued that not all states face the same security threats, therefore one cannot exogenously presume a state's security interests (Youde, 2004, p. 194). This model of securitisation theory makes the concept of security more relevant to meeting security challenges such as HIV-AIDS and Ebola. Although preferring the term 'biosecurity', David Fidler and Lawrence Gostin (2008, p. 9) posit that security is impossible without closer integration of the health and security communities. Writing from the Asian SARS experience, Caballero-Anthony iterates "the threats of infectious diseases require urgent responses. The regional community and states need not wait for the worst-case scenario of state failure before infectious diseases can be considered as a matter of national security. Hence, there is a need to securitise" (Caballero-Anthony, 2005, p. 489). This suggests that the traditionalists' focus on military threats alone is superficial; here, the threat of SARS is considered a national security issue threatening complete state failure. This underscores Fidler and Lawrence's (2008) argument that security is impossible without integrating health into the discourse. Additionally, it can be argued that elevating health issues to the level of security concerns offers opportunities to mobilise greater political force and key resources to address a variety of global health issues.

However, some scholars and policy makers have cast doubt about the influence and utility of conflating health and security concerns. It can be argued that responding to health issues as national security threats transforms the logic of international health action into one based on narrow states' self-interests, corresponding to the traditional concept of security where state survival takes precedence. Thus, arguably, the securitisation concept gives precedence to the security of states and considers international health policies as instruments in pursuit of national security (McInnes & Rushton, 2012). For instance, the UK and US governments have perceived global health engagement as state security ends. The White House, in 2009, endorsed President Obama's Global Health Initiative as an "important component of the national security 'smart power' strategy" (The White House, 2009). Similarly, the UK government's Global Health Report for 2008 depicts Global Health Initiatives as instruments to pursue national security (HM Government, 2008). Consequently, global health policies tend to exhibit focuses on pragmatism rather than humanitarianism; and cannot deliver effective health schemes focused on human wellbeing (McInnes & Rushton, 2012), as health policies become a means to realise state ends.

The instrumental perception of global health security conjures questions about conceptual and normative appropriateness. Viewing health through the lenses of state interest creates imbalanced prioritisation of global health: communicable diseases potentially threatening state security receive greater attention and resources than non-communicable and chronic conditions (Davis, 2010). Despite being critical health issues for many individuals, non-communicable diseases such as diarrheal diseases, killing 1.8 million annually of which 90% are children (McInnes & Lee, 2006, p. 11), receive little attention from a securitisation perspective. Successful securitisation of health issues advances beyond routine political discourse, prioritising them atop political agendas and giving them maximum attention and resources (Davis, 2010). Essentially, one concern of securitising global health issues is that they only become a 'crisis' when Western countries feel threatened (Roemer-Mahler & Rushton, 2016, p. 375), suggesting that securitisation process is selective and, arguably, Eurocentric. This was evidenced when the US 2002 National Security Strategy inferred that 'good governance' should be a condition for health aid, signifying human access to better health is not a 'necessity', but subordinate to neoliberal Western ideas of democracy (McInnes & Lee, 2006). This approach could create inaction or inadequate responses to tackling deadly diseases that do not pose security threats to the West.

Furthermore, global health security literature predominantly favours a negative version of security, whereby security is understood as security from existential threat (Brown & Stoeva, 2014, p. 306), adopting the traditional view of security as survival (Booth, 2007). Conversely, a positive version of security covers the pursuit of individual wellbeing as a means of achieving long-term stability and security (Gjorv, 2012). Security theories which promote a negative conception of security construct an understanding of health purely as survival and security from threats. Yet, health is far more than freedom from disease or survival: people can survive free from diseases, yet live in very poor sanitation or lack adequate nourishment, which would not constitute healthy living. While critics argue that poor sanitation, for instance, does not conform to security as existential threat, securitising health only on the premise of 'existential threat' shifts the focus from the individual as the referent object to the state, reinforcing the realist conception of security. This approach is problematic, because state security then takes precedence over human health, by addressing health issues that threaten the state rather than health issues that threaten human life. Accordingly, this negative conceptualisation of security tends to isolate health from its systemic causes and favour responsive rather than preventative strategies.

Research papers presented at the Centre for Global Health Policy expose further limitations of health securitisation: framing global health issues as technical biomedical conundrums to either be prevented or cured, failing to mitigate the principal structures that create and reproduce global health inequalities (Anderson, 2014; Nunes, 2016). This suggests that predominant focus is on the technicalities of diseases, instead of the political environment. In evidence, Yassif et al. (2013) note that a Chatham House report outlined recommendations for disease prevention that focus exclusively on the problems posed by "potentially threatening bio-technology and human-animal contact" (Jegat, 2015, p. 3). The risk of framing global health as a technical biomedical challenge is that it both shifts focus from the underlying political structures, and hampers long term developmental projects to potentially enhance both human and state security.

Responses to the recent Ebola outbreak in West Africa typify these explanations. Attention paid to the virus was episodic, temporary, and arose from concerns with countering an outbreak that potentially constituted a threat to national security, unambiguously to the West (Davies, 2015). This paper concentrates next on the Ebola response in West Africa.

Understanding the Ebola Response in West Africa: Background

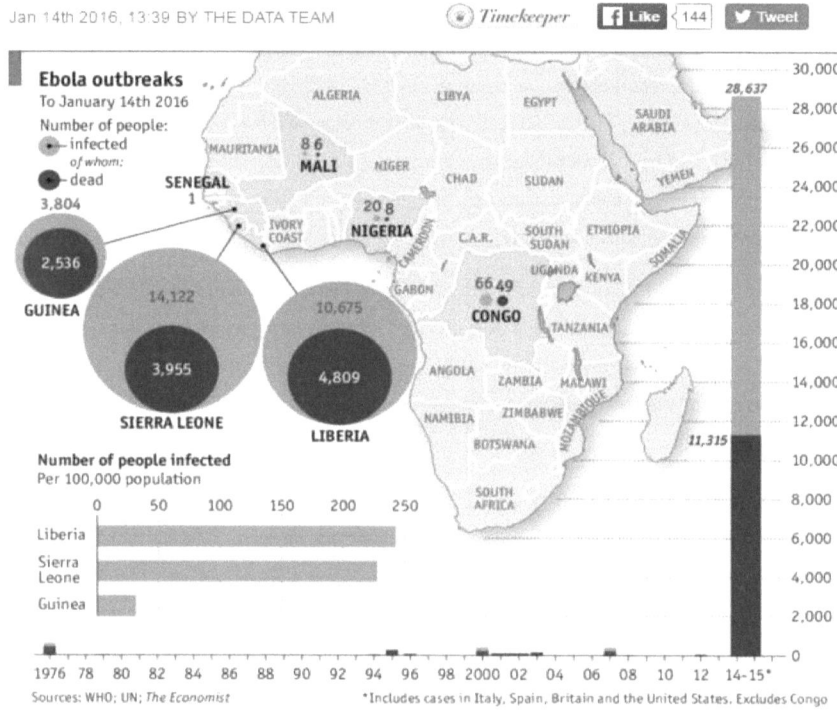

Figure 1: Ebola Daily Chart   **Source: The Economist (2016)**

The World Health Organisation (WHO) in January 2016 declared Africa, particularly Liberia, Guinea, and Sierra Leone, free of the deadly Ebola killer virus. In December 2013, the first reported case occurred in a remote area of Guinea, near the border with Liberia and Sierra Leone. By the end of March 2014, Liberia and Sierra Leone reported suspected cases of eight and six respectively, owing to cross-border migration with Guinea. By June 2014, 467 people had died out of 759 reported cases (The Economist, 2016). By January 14 2016, a total of 28,637 cases and 11, 315 deaths had been reported worldwide with Liberia, Guinea, and Sierra Leone recording 99.87% of the casualties (The Economist, 2016), illustrated by Figure 1. The ensuing section analyses how the pandemic evolved from 'a West African problem' to a Western problem, constructing the pandemic as a national security threat.

From a West African Problem to a Western Problem

The Ebola virus disease (EVD) was named after the Congolese river Ebola in a rural region of the former Zaire, now the Democratic Republic of Congo (DRC), where it was first identified in 1976. Prior to 2014, Uganda recorded the largest outbreak in 2000, in which 425 were infected and 224 died (Renwick, 2016). Therefore, the pandemic, including its mode of transmission, symptoms, and deadly nature, was not unknown to the global community. Yet, the deadly Ebola pandemic in West Africa was not perceived as an 'existential threat' requiring an emergency response, despite calculations showing that 3 in every 5 reported cases died during the first half of 2014 (The Economist, 2016). Even when Doctors Without Borders (MSF), a nongovernmental organisation, deployed doctors into the three West African countries and described the situation on the ground as "unprecedented" in March 2014, international organisations, including WHO, and foreign governments only declared a health emergency in August 2014. The obvious timing question is answered by the death from Ebola of an American citizen in Nigeria who travelled from Liberia at the end of July 2014 (Wilson, 2014). His death in a Nigerian hospital set off a chain of transmission that infected 19 people and caused 7 deaths in Nigeria (WHO, WHO declares end of Ebola outbreak in Nigeria, 2014). Additionally, further US victims of the Ebola virus, Dr Kent Brantly and Nancy Writebol, working in Christian missions in Liberia were respectively flown to the US on August 2nd and 5th (McClam & Chuck, 2014).

Prior to US citizens becoming infected with the virus, the UK's Chief Medical Officer, Dame Sally Davies, dismissed a call by security analysts to implement safety procedures between infected countries and the UK and to take action against the deadly pandemic in West Africa, claiming: "there had been no reports of cases having been 'exported' to countries outside of West Africa. Airport screenings, the letter implied, were 'costly' and could be expected to have 'limited impact' given that the virus has an incubation period of 21 days" (Rodrigues, 2014). However, following the cases involving US citizens, the UK Foreign Secretary Philip Hammond summoned an emergency Cobra meeting which recognised that Ebola was not just a West African problem, and thus threatened UK national security if action was not taken to stop the spread of the virus in West Africa (Rodrigues, 2014). Similarly, President Obama declared the Ebola outbreak as a national security priority for the United States. Accordingly, WHO called a two-day emergency meeting after which it announced, on August 8, that the Ebola epidemic in West Africa is an 'extraordinary event' and thus constituted a global health risk. The Geneva-based UN agency added that *"a coordinated international response is deemed essential to stop and reverse the international spread of Ebola"* (Kelland, 2014, citing WHO).

At this point there was a persuasive appeal by WHO that an existential threat existed requiring an emergency response, and a global audience who accepted this claim by the securitising actor, WHO.

However, the justification to *'stop and reverse international spread of Ebola'* signifies that the objective was stopping the spread of Ebola outside West Africa's borders, rather than saving human lives. In effect, the call for intervention was for state security, not human security, reasons. Also, the failure by WHO to 'securitise' Ebola, even when the West African death-survival ratio was 3:5, underscores the assertion that the securitisation process is selective and Eurocentric: WHO's two-day emergency meeting was convened only days after US citizens became casualties and were flown to the US. This raises the question whether the Ebola outbreak would have undergone the securitisation process if there were no Western casualties. The next section discusses the global response to the Ebola outbreak in Guinea, Liberia, and Sierra Leone.

Global Response

Despite the outbreak's rapid rates of infection and death, the international community had been slow to respond. In September 2014, following the August securitisation Ebola, donor countries, led by the United Kingdom, France, and the USA, declared their commitment to tackle the deadly virus. However, historical links determined how direct foreign aid was distributed: "The United States led relief efforts in Liberia, which was founded by freed U.S. slaves, and the United Kingdom and France led efforts in their former colonies Sierra Leone and Guinea, respectively" (Renwick, 2016). By the first quarter of 2015, the US and the UK had deployed military personnel to provide medical and logistics support to the various West African countries. Financially, more than \$8.2 billion was pledged by individual donors, institutions and countries (see Appendix 1).

However, the rapid outbreak of the EVD in the three West African countries should not be seen merely as an aid problem, but rather a symptom of a weak health care system. Given that the three infected countries are still recovering from protracted civil wars, aid and health assistance are, nevertheless, essential as resources are rationed for already strained budgets and health departments. There is an overall lack of adequate trained medical personnel, basic kits, and suitable healthcare facilities to cope with the demands on healthcare. For instance, research shows that Liberia which has a population of more than four million people had less than 50 doctors working in the public health system prior to the Ebola crisis (Farmer, 2014, pp. 38-39). This suggests that there is 1 doctor to every 100,000 people, compared to 670 doctors to every 100,000 in Cuba, and 240 doctors to every 100,000 in the US (Farmer, 2014). Therefore, the securitisation paradigm, which tends to conceptualise global health security via the prism of state interests, has consequentially directed substantial amount of resources to stopping the spread of Ebola only as a responsive mechanism, ignoring its systemic causes, as well as failing to deal with the structural causes of global health inequalities that produce and reproduce these pandemics. In evidence, as stated earlier, Ebola is a symptom of a weak healthcare system and its "ability to spread was largely due to the stricken countries' weak health-care systems" (Renwick,

2016): Nigeria and US, for example, were able to stop the pandemic's potency to spread in their countries due to their relatively stronger medical systems. This also implies that securitisation discourse only provides temporary emergency measures to global health issues instead of permanent health security solutions.

Not only was Ebola framed as a national security priority, but as a biomedical problem. President Obama in a speech described the pandemic as a "biomedical danger" (Levine, 2014), a "challenge to inventors and entrepreneurs and businesses of the world" (Levine, 2014) to produce protective equipment to combat the disease. The problem with framing Ebola as a technical biomedical challenge is that it fails to address the existing health inequalities in Guinea, Liberia and Sierra Leone. It can be argued that securitising Ebola in 2014 merely acted as a pull for government officials in these three countries to acquire further resources for downwards distribution, owing to patron-client relations, in exchange for loyalty (Jegat, 2015, p. 3). The risk of framing Ebola as a technical biomedical challenge is not only potentially diverting focus from the underlying political structures in the impacted countries, but additionally hindering long term developmental projects designed to enhance both human security and state security, while benefitting "elites at the top of the neo-patrimonial structure" (Jegat, 2015, p. 3).

Ebola Mitigation Measures

Securitisation of health, reliant on emergency response control measures, implies there was no available pharmaceutical solution to combat a deadly disease like Ebola, despite being known to global health policy makers for years. Accordingly, containment strategies were adopted to mitigate the rapid outbreak of the disease in Liberia, Guinea and Sierra Leone: case isolation, quarantine, and sanitary funeral practices were implemented with "utmost urgency" in the quest to reverse the epidemic's spread (Pandey et al., 2014). Isolation involves a controlled avoidance of any contact with the outer world for a defined period, in this case for 21 days, after coming in contact with an Ebola patient; quarantine requires compulsory isolation of the Ebola patient from any contact with the outer world, with professional monitoring. Whereas rapid containment strategies were argued to have been successful in previous Ebola outbreaks, WHO has reported that the strategies failed to work in Guinea, Liberia and Sierra Leone, due to lack of capacity and insufficient healthcare workers in these countries' dysfunctional healthcare systems: "Some treatment facilities are overflowing; all beds are occupied and patients are being turned away. Many facilities lack reliable supplies of electricity and running water" (WHO, 2014). This illustrates that securitisation, together with its emergency and temporary response measures, are inadequate to deal with global and public health issues such as Ebola.

Considering the previous limited outbreaks of Ebola in the DRC, Uganda et cetera, one might expect diagnostic tools and vaccines were prioritised and developed by WHO during the inter-epidemic periods to accelerate development and intervention when similar outbreaks re-occur. This failure underscores the argument of many scholars that global and public health governance should consider pharmaceuticalisation as a step in the right direction to countering global health threats (Abraham, 2010; Elbe, 2010). Acquiring medical countermeasures in the form of antibiotics, antivirals, anti-toxins, and next-generation vaccines, could help stop the devastating outbreak of such epidemics, and in this case, Ebola.

Conclusion

This paper has critically analysed the Copenhagen School's securitisation model. As a speech act discourse, securitisation theory has contributed considerably to understanding security in international relations. The paper has argued that the Copenhagen School's conceptualisation of global security favours a 'negative' version of security, understanding security as security from existential threat, supporting the traditional conception of security as survival. This isolates health issues from their systemic causes, instigating responsive mechanisms rather than preventative policies, and fails to deal with the structural causes of global health producing and reproducing these pandemics. Accordingly, the issues of human wellbeing and the systemic causes of ill health receive inadequate focus. The study has also argued that this approach to conceptualising security conjures the understanding of health via the prism of state interests, as communicable diseases are perceived to pose potential threats to state security. Subsequently, substantial attention and resources are directed towards communicable, rather than non-communicable and chronic, diseases. The paper has drawn on the recent Ebola outbreak largely in Guinea, Liberia and Sierra Leone to substantiate the arguments, revealing that the propensity to focus on standard containment measures obscured long-term background factors: inadequate health infrastructure and insufficient domestic health workers. This exacerbated the transmission of Ebola and ensured the virus was not effectively identified in its early stages. The long term delivery of effective global health policy requires a preventative rather than reactive approach, with a focus on strengthening the domestic health capacity of states (Davies, 2015). While emergency responses may effectively contain disease outbreaks, a preoccupation with quarantine and containment measures rather than building long-term domestic health capacity means that global health strategies will continually be responding to disease outbreaks rather than preventing them. Another potential approach is the pharmaceuticalisation of global health proposed by some public health scholars.

4017 words

Bibliography

Abraham, J. (2010). Pharmaceuticalization of society in context: theoretical, empirical and health dimensions. *Sociology, 44*(4), 603-622. doi:10.1177/0038038510369368

Anderson, E.-L. (2014). Health Systems Subverting and the Ebola Crisis', 'The Ebola Crisis: An International Relations Response? *Centre for Global Health Policy.* University of Sussex.

Austin, J. (1962). *How to do things with words.* Cambridge: Harvard University Press.

Booth. (2007). *Theory of World Security.* Cambridge: Cambridge University Press.

Brown, G., & Stoeva, P. (2014). An ounce of prevention is worth a pound of cure: reevaluating health security from a cosmopolitan perspective. In S. Rushton, & J. Youde (Eds.), *Routledge Handbook of Global Health Security* (pp. 304-317). London: Routledge.

Buzan, B., Waever, O., & de Wilde, J. (1998). *Security: A new framework for analysis.* Boulder: Lynne Rienner.

Caballero-Anthony, M. (2005). SARS in Asia: Crisis, Vulnerabilities, and Regional Responses. *Asian Survey, 45*(3), 475-495.

Davies, S. (2015). *Ebola Outbreak: Politics of Prevention and Engagement.* Retrieved from Australian Institute of International Affairs: http://www.internationalaffairs.org.au/australian_outlook/ebola-outbreak-politics-of-prevention-and-engagement/

Davis, S. (2010). *Global Politics of Health.* Cambridge: Polity Press.

Elbe, S. (2010). *Security and Global Health.* Cambridge: Polity Press.

Farmer, P. (2014). Diary. *London Review of Books, 36*(20), 38-39.

Fidler, D., & Gostin, L. (2008). *Biosecurity in Global Age: Biological Weapons, Public Health and the Rule of Law.* Palo Alto, Calif.: Stanford University Press.

Gjorv, G. (2012). Security by any other name: negative security, positive security and a multi-actor security approach. *Review of International Studies, 38*(4), 835-859.

HM Government. (2008). *Health is Global: an outcomes framework for global health 2011-15.* Retrieved from HM Government: https://www.gov.uk/government/uploads/system/uploads/attachment_data/file/67578/health-is-global.pdf

Jegat, J. (2015, November 17). *Global Pandemics: A Security Threat?* Retrieved from E-international relations: http://www.e-ir.info/2015/11/17/global-pandemics-a-security-threat/

Kelland, K. (2014, August 8). *WHO declares Ebola epidemic an international health emergency.* Retrieved from Reuters: http://www.reuters.com/article/us-health-ebola-emergency-idUSKBN0G80M620140808

Levine, S. (2014, September 26). *Obama: Ebola a 'security priority'.* Retrieved from Politico: http://www.politico.com/story/2014/09/obama-ebola-global-health-security-agenda-summit-111355

McClam, E., & Chuck, E. (2014, October 24th). *Ebola in America: The State of the Virus in the U.S.* Retrieved from NBC News: http://www.nbcnews.com/storyline/ebola-virus-outbreak/ebola-america-state-virus-u-s-n228426

McInnes, C., & Lee, K. (2006). Health, security and foreign policy. *Review of International Studies, 32*(1), 5-23. doi:10.1017/S0260210506006905

McInnes, C., & Rushton, S. (2012). Smart Power? Health interventions for strategic effect in Iraq and Afghanistan. *International Political Sociology, 6*(3), 328-331.

Nunes, J. (2016). Ebola and the production of neglect in global health. *Third World Quarterly, 37*(3), 542-556. doi:10.1080/01436597.2015.1124724

O'Neill, O. (2002). Public Health or Clinical Ethics: Thinking beyond borders. *Ethics & International Affairs, 16*(2), 35-45.

Pandey et al. (2014). Strategies for containing Ebola in West Africa. *Science, 346*(6212), 991-995. doi:10.1126/science.1260612

Renwick, D. (2016, January 15). *Ebola Virus*. Retrieved from Council on Foreign Relations: http://www.cfr.org/africa-sub-saharan/ebola-virus/p33661

Rodrigues, C. (2014, August 6). *The world must wake up: Ebola outbreak is not just a West African problem*. Retrieved from New Internationalist Magazine: http://newint.org/features/web-exclusive/2014/08/06/ebola-international-response/

Roemer-Mahler, A., & Rushton, S. (2016). Introduction: Ebola and International Relations. *Third World Quarterly, 37*(3), 373-379. doi:10.1080/01436597.2015.1118343

The Economist. (2016, January 14). *Ebola in Africa: the end of a tragedy?* Retrieved from The Economist: http://www.economist.com/blogs/graphicdetail/2016/01/daily-chart-12

The White House. (2009, May 5). *Statement by the President on Global Health Initiative*. Retrieved from The White House: https://www.whitehouse.gov/the-press-office/statement-president-global-health-initiative

Waever, O. (1995). Securitization and Desecuritization. In R. Lipschutz (Ed.), *On Security* (pp. 46-86). New York: Columbia University Press.

WHO. (2014, August 11). *Emergencies preparedness, response: Barriers to rapid containment of the Ebola outbreak*. Retrieved from World Health Organization: http://www.who.int/csr/disease/ebola/overview-august-2014/en/

WHO. (2014, October 20). *WHO declares end of Ebola outbreak in Nigeria*. Retrieved from World Health Organisation: http://www.who.int/mediacentre/news/statements/2014/nigeria-ends-ebola/en/

Williams, M. C. (2003). Words, Images, Enemies: Securitization and International Politics. *International Studies Quarterly, 47*(4), 511–531. doi:10.1046/j.0020-8833.2003.00277.x

Wilson, J. (2014, July 30). *Ebola fears hit close to home: Ebola outbreak kills an American*. Retrieved from CNN: http://edition.cnn.com/2014/07/29/health/ebola-outbreak-american-dies/

World Bank. (2015, 10 14). *Global Ebola Response - Resource Tracking (Work in Progress)*. Retrieved from World Bank:

http://pubdocs.worldbank.org/pubdocs/publicdoc/2015/10/224781444934423554/World-
Banks-Global-Ebola-Response-Resource-Tracking-as-of-10-14-15.pdf

Youde, J. (2004, March 17-20). *Enter the Fourth Horseman: Health Security and International
Relations Theory*. Retrieved from Researchgate:
https://www.researchgate.net/publication/237497080_Enter_the_Fourth_Horseman_Healt
h_Security_and_International_Relations_Theory

Appendix 1

Global Ebola Response - Resource Tracking (Work in Progress)

As of 10/14/2015

 Note: all amounts represent US$ x 1,000 unless otherwise

Source:

http://pubdocs.worldbank.org/pubdocs/publicdoc/2015/10/224781444934423554/World-Banks-Global-Ebola-Response-Resource-Tracking-as-of-10-14-15.pdf

Please see document on the next page.

Global Ebola Response - Resource Tracking (Work in Progress)

As of 10/14/2015

(note: all amounts represent US$ x 1,000 unless otherwise specified)

Pledge
A non-binding announcement of an intended contribution or allocation by the donor

DONOR/COUNTRY	Guinea	Liberia	Sierra Leone	Total (3 Countries: Guinea + Liberia + Sleone)	Other Countries	Supranational (regional/subregional allocations)	Non Country Specific Pledges	Cumulative Total Pledges by Donor As Of 10/14/2015
UNITED STATES	129,146	1,027,091	155,384	1,311,621	703,486	69,206	-	2,084,313
WORLD BANK GROUP	260,000	385,000	318,000	963,000	-	69,300	585,700	1,618,000
EUROPEAN COMMISSION	216,088	210,674	246,130	672,892	35,200	247,286	-	955,378
UNITED KINGDOM	-	1,180	324,000	325,180	-	-	362,133	687,313
AFRICAN DEVELOPMENT BANK	51,600	77,000	81,000	209,600	12,467	1,000	302,300	525,367
GERMANY	55,833	52,984	54,124	162,941	-	17,091	265,935	445,967
INTERNATIONAL MONETARY FUND	132,700	130,100	140,800	403,600	-	-	-	403,600
FRANCE	145,927	-	-	145,927	-	26,532	92,863	265,322
JAPAN	11,090	14,009	9,470	34,569	-	-	138,420	172,989
CHINA	-	-	-	-	-	123,000	6,000	129,000
CANADA	10,052	5,044	1,227	16,323	2,391	15,600	80,897	115,211
PAUL ALLEN FOUNDATION	-	6,600	-	6,600	-	93,400	-	100,000
NETHERLANDS	4,054	3,716	5,135	12,905	-	2,980	67,047	82,932
SWEDEN	1,289	8,672	4,032	13,994	222	49,947	16,571	80,734
NORWAY	-	-	-	-	-	63,475	-	63,475
RUSSIAN FEDERATION	-	-	-	-	-	-	55,100	55,100
BILL & MELINDA GATES FOUNDATION	500	4,000	2,333	6,833	6,360	17,085	24,191	54,469
BELGIUM	-	-	-	-	-	-	50,934	50,934
AUSTRALIA	-	-	19,826	19,826	-	4,957	13,067	37,850
SAUDI ARABIA	-	-	-	-	-	-	35,000	35,000
DENMARK	-	-	5,100	5,100	3,400	13,510	10,200	32,210
SPECIAL RELIEF FUND	-	-	-	-	-	-	28,500	28,500
MARK ZUCKERBERG & PRISCILLA CHAN	-	-	-	-	-	25,000	-	25,000
ISLAMIC DEVELOPMENT BANK	5,419	-	300	5,719	-	-	10,000	15,719
FINLAND	-	-	-	-	-	-	13,265	13,265
KOREA	-	-	-	-	-	-	12,600	12,600
INDIA	50	50	50	150	-	-	12,050	12,200
AGENCE FRANCAISE DE DEVELOPMENT	-	-	-	-	10,575	-	-	10,575
SWITZERLAND	-	-	-	-	-	-	9,832	9,832
ITALY	-	-	9,148	9,148	253	307	-	9,709
BRAZIL	-	-	-	-	-	-	9,626	9,626
ISRAEL	-	-	-	-	-	-	8,750	8,750
IRELAND	33	1,299	4,668	6,001	-	-	1,521	7,521
IKEA FOUNDATION	-	133	-	133	-	6,633	-	6,765
THE PRUDENTIAL FOUNDATION	-	-	-	-	-	-	6,700	6,700
KUWAIT	-	-	-	-	-	-	5,000	5,000
NIGERIA	-	-	-	-	-	-	5,000	5,000
VENEZUELA	-	-	-	-	-	-	5,000	5,000
NEW ZEALAND	-	-	1,659	1,659	-	-	2,488	4,147
AUSTRIA	663	663	1,021	2,348	1,327	-	-	3,675
PHILIPPINES	-	-	-	-	-	-	2,000	2,000
TIMOR LESTE	-	-	2,000	2,000	-	-	-	2,000
AZERBAIJAN	-	-	-	-	-	-	1,000	1,000
BOLIVIA	-	-	-	-	-	-	1,000	1,000
COTE D'IVOIRE	-	-	-	-	-	-	1,000	1,000
NAMIBIA	-	-	-	-	-	-	1,000	1,000
Cumulative Pledges by Country	1,024,445	1,928,216	1,385,408	4,338,069	775,681	846,308	2,242,692	8,202,749

*

The World Bank tracks Ebola resource flows (including monetized in-kind contributions where available) totaling US$1 million or more from multilateral and bilateral institutions and some foundations. Data is captured from government and other official websites and from communication with key officials within development partner agencies. Data is updated on a monthly basis. Pledges are a non-binding announcement of an intended contribution or allocation by the donor.
To report pledge information, please contact Viji Iyer at viyer@worldbank.org

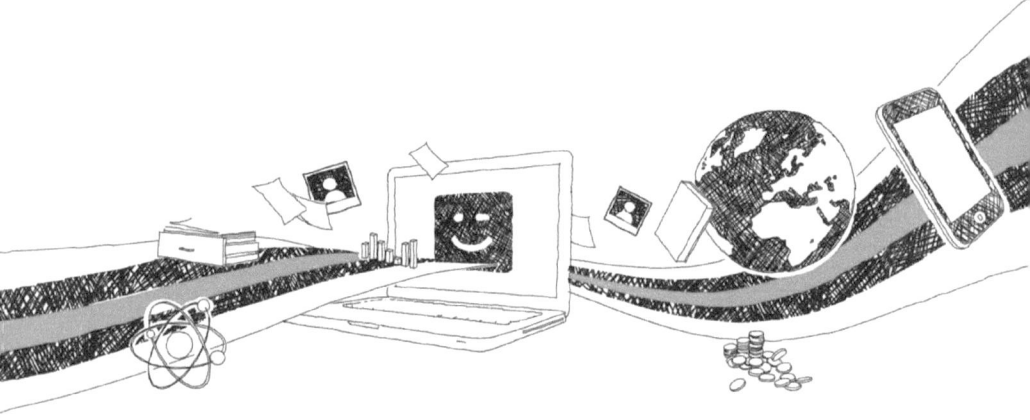
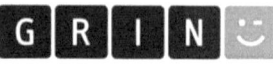